Plan for Success

12-Week Meal & Lifestyle Journal

The Essential WLS Companion

This Journal Belongs to

_____

Plan for Success

12-Week Meal & Lifestyle Journal

The Essential WLS Companion

A success-promoting tool for people that want to lose weight and maintain a healthy weight after bariatric surgery.

A LIVINGAFTERWLS PUBLICATION

Proudly serving the weight loss surgery community since 2005.

ISBN-13: 978-1708724009

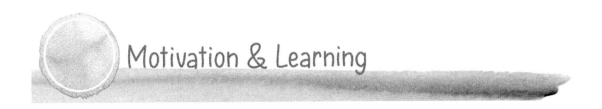

Letter from Kaye

It was two decades ago -*September 1999*- that I had gastric bypass surgery. Most 20-year-old surgeries are nothing but a vague memory and a faded scar. Not weight loss surgery. It is part of my day, every day. Most days I feel robust enthusiasm for life. Occasionally I have days when I question my sanity 20 years ago when I opted for surgery. Do you ever ask yourself, "What the hell was I thinking?" We have all been there, I think.

Managing a healthy weight with WLS is a challenge that I certainly underestimated. It is not the "easy way out" as the ignorant often describe it. I have found my best days are when I've planned my meals –*even a jotted note is better than leaving things to chance*- and held myself accountable. Planning, goal setting, accountability. This is the function of a dedicated planner or journal such as this 12-Week Planner. Thank you for making it a part of your WLS journey: I hope you find it as valuable as I do.

Not Vanity: Weight management is not owned by vanity. It is a matter of life and death. We must buckle down and accept the challenge to continue fighting the disease with fierce passion. Bariatric surgery is the most effective treatment of obesity and the secondary diseases associated with it. WLS is known to produce long-lasting health benefits. But the surgery does not work alone. It is our battle to win and victory can only be accomplished by understanding, accepting, and living by the rules.

It behooves us to develop strategies for navigating in the real world. When we have surgery, we changed and then we returned to the exact environment we lived in prior to surgery: the very environment that contributed to our obesity. We can enjoy lasting success with surgery when we evolve strategies for navigating our new body in the old waters.

You are not alone! I wish you splendid life-long health and wellness in your journey with WLS.

Kaye Bailey
LivingAfterWLS Founder, Patient mentor & advocate, gastric bypass patient

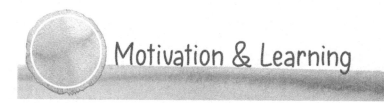

Make a Plan, Not a Wish

Simply not wanting to be overweight is a wish, not a plan.

One way to motivate yourself is to recognize how gratifying it is to make a commitment to a goal, identify the specific steps to get there, follow your plan, and reap the rewards

Quarterly Personal Self-Assessment

Date:

The LivingAfterWLS "Quarterly Personal Self-Assessment" tool is a worksheet of questions we can ask ourselves in a sincere effort to assess our present state and make an action plan for the next three months. This worksheet should be used as a private tool with the intent to keep your eye on the goal. It is a contract with yourself; a contract of honor and self-respect because you deserve to treat yourself well and engage in appropriate long-term behaviors in pursuit of your healthiest life. Please accept this invitation to join me in the Quarterly Personal Self-Assessment. Take some quiet time to evaluate where you are and where you are going. Commit your WLS goals to paper. Pre-ops, Newbies and Old-timers all benefit from the use of this tool. You can do this. *Always review your previous quarterly worksheets as you begin this exercise.*

_ _

Body: I am physically WELL/ILL *and this is supporting/disrupting my healthy efforts.*

I weigh _____ and I'm [ ] LOSING [ ] GAINING [ ] MAINTAINING.

Mind: I am mentally FOCUSED/DISTRACTED *regarding my WLS experience.*

> *My thoughts are:*

Heart: I am socially and emotionally HAPPY/SAD which is positively/negatively affecting my well-being.

> *My relationships are:*

Write a personal assessment briefly summarizing your overall health and wellness pertaining specifically to your obesity management with weight loss surgery:

My top three goals when I had WLS were:

> Indicate if they are ONGOING (O) CHANGED (C) or ACHIEVED (A)
> 1)
> 2)
> 3)

In pursuit of these goals list the strengths and strategies that are contributing to favorable results:

As with any journey there are struggles. Where have you struggled and what improvements could be made to produce better results?

Define the goal you will pursue this quarter. Why is it important and worthy of your energy and effort? Does it contribute to your long-term health and weight management?

Including your strengths, knowledge, abilities, and intentions define your approach to achieving this goal. Map a strategy for each barrier.

Make a commitment.
Based on the assessment above I will:

The specific tools/methods I will use for my success are:

Will I enlist the help of others? Who/What:

Make your agreement binding:
My next appointment for self-assessment is: _____ (see page 135)

In solemn contract with myself I hereby agree to honor these commitments:

_____

Signature & Date

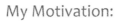

Tracking & Progress

I've got this!

My concerns:

My Motivation:

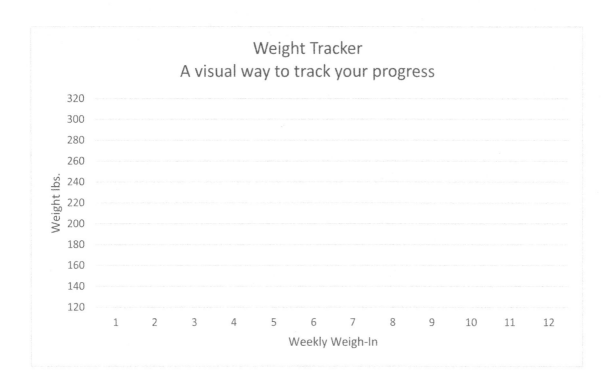

Weight Tracker
A visual way to track your progress

Weight lbs.

320
300
280
260
240
220
200
180
160
140
120

1   2   3   4   5   6   7   8   9   10   11   12

Weekly Weigh-In

THE BIG PICTURE:

Based on my Self-Assessment for the next 12 weeks my health and wellness objectives are:

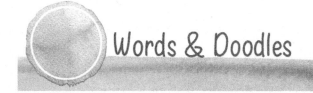

Words & Doodles

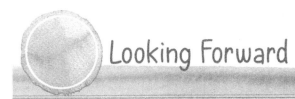

Looking Forward

Month/Year

SUNDAY	MONDAY	TUESDAY	WEDNESDAY	THURSDAY	FRIDAY	SATURDAY

Obstacle Awareness:
Mindful Preparedness

Words & Doodles

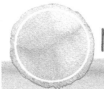

New Week: Great Plan

Protein First Meals

Monday	
Tuesday	
Wednesday	
Thursday	
Friday	
Saturday	
Sunday	

Week 1: Goals

Take a small step to improve your health through diet, fitness, and behavior. Add something; eliminate something; change a habit; try something new.
For each category show: ACTION/REWARD

Diet & Nutrition

/
/

Activities of Living

Physical movement in the daily routine

/
/

Fitness Exercise

Activity for the purpose of health

/
/

Notes:

Grocery List

○ ○ ○ ○
○ ○ ○ ○
○ ○ ○ ○
○ ○ ○ Budget $
○ ○ ○ Actual: $

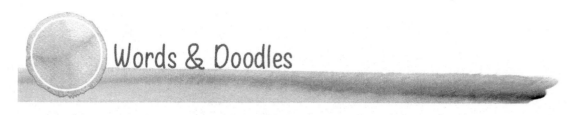

The Four Rules of WLS

Protein First: At every meal the WLS patient will eat lean animal, dairy, or vegetable protein before any other food. Protein shakes or supplements may be included as part of the weight loss surgery diet. Patients are advised to consume 60-105 grams of protein a day. Eating lean protein will create a tight feeling in the surgical stomach pouch: this feeling is the signal to stop eating. Many patients report discomfort when eating lean protein, yet this discomfort is the very reason the stomach pouch is effective in reducing food and caloric intake. Animal products are the most nutrient rich source of protein and include fish, shellfish, poultry, and meat. Dairy protein, including eggs, yogurt, and cheese, is another excellent source of protein.

Lots of Water: Like most weight loss plans bariatric surgery patients are instructed to drink lots of water throughout the day. Most centers advise a minimum of 64 fluid ounces of water each day. Water hydrates the organs and cells and facilitates the metabolic processes of human life. Water flushes toxins and waste from the body. Patients are strongly discouraged from drinking carbonated beverages. In addition, patients are warned against excessive alcohol intake as it tends to have a quicker and more profound intoxicating affect compared with pre-surgery consumption. In addition, non-nutritional beverages of any kind may lead to weight gain and increased snacking.

No Snacking: Patients are discouraged from snacking which may impede weight loss and lead to weight gain. Specifically, patients are forbidden to partake of traditional processed carbohydrate snacks, such as chips, crackers, baked goods, and sweets. Patients who return to snacking on empty calorie non-nutritional food defeat the restrictive nature of the surgery and weight gain results. It is seemingly contradictory that the 5DPT allows snacking. High protein snacks are allowed because they keep the metabolism active, they satiate hunger, and they help relieve the symptoms of carbohydrate withdrawal.

Daily Exercise: In general patients are advised to engage in 30 minutes of physical activity on most days of the week. The most effective way to heal the body from the ravages of obesity is to exercise. Exercise means moving the body: walking, stretching, bending, inhaling and exhaling. Exercise is the most effective, most enjoyable, most beneficial gift one can receive when recovering from life threatening, crippling morbid obesity. Consistent exercise will keep morbid obesity in remission and help compensate for lapses in following the three other rules. People who successfully maintain their weight exercise daily.

Notes:

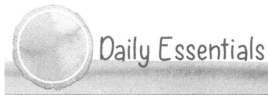
Daily Essentials

Today Is:
S M T W T F S

Protein First Meals
Protein goal: grams/day

Morning	PRO	CARBS	FAT	CALORIES
Midday	PRO	CARBS	FAT	CALORIES
Evening	PRO	CARBS	FAT	CALORIES
Protein Snack	PRO	CARBS	FAT	CALORIES
Beverages				

Today's Energy Intake
PRO   CARBS   FAT   CALORIES

Obstacle Awareness:
Mindful Preparedness

Daily Activities
ACTIVITY/DURATION
Fitness Exercise
Activity for the purpose of health

/

Activities of Living
Physical movement in the daily routine

/

Extra Mile
Intentional physical activity beyond the necessary:
taking stairs, walking vs. transport; standing vs.
sitting; etc.

/

Today I was active for:

___Hour ____ Min

Emoji of the Day

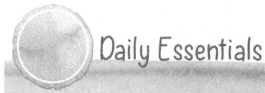 # Daily Essentials

Today Is:
S M T W T F S

Protein First Meals
Protein goal: grams/day

Morning			
	PRO CARBS FAT CALORIES		
Midday			
	PRO CARBS FAT CALORIES		
Evening			
	PRO CARBS FAT CALORIES		
Protein Snack			
	PRO CARBS FAT CALORIES		
Beverages			

Today's Energy Intake
PRO   CARBS   FAT   CALORIES

Obstacle Awareness:
Mindful Preparedness

Daily Activities
ACTIVITY/DURATION

Fitness Exercise
Activity for the purpose of health

/

Activities of Living
Physical movement in the daily routine

/

Extra Mile
Intentional physical activity beyond the necessary: taking stairs, walking vs. transport; standing vs. sitting; etc.

/

Today I was active for:

___Hour_____Min

Emoji of the Day
☺ 😐 🙂 ☹ ◯

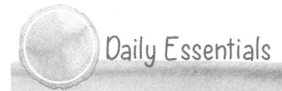 Daily Essentials

Protein First Meals
Protein goal: grams/day

Morning			
PRO	CARBS	FAT	CALORIES
Midday			
PRO	CARBS	FAT	CALORIES
Evening			
PRO	CARBS	FAT	CALORIES
Protein Snack			
PRO	CARBS	FAT	CALORIES

Beverages

Today's Energy Intake
PRO   CARBS   FAT   CALORIES

Obstacle Awareness:
Mindful Preparedness

Daily Activities
ACTIVITY/DURATION

Fitness Exercise
Activity for the purpose of health

/

Activities of Living
Physical movement in the daily routine

/

Extra Mile
Intentional physical activity beyond the necessary: taking stairs, walking vs. transport; standing vs. sitting; etc.

/

Today I was active for:

___Hour ____ Min

Emoji of the Day

Daily Essentials

Protein First Meals
Protein goal: grams/day

Obstacle Awareness: Mindful Preparedness

Morning				
	PRO	CARBS	FAT	CALORIES

Midday				
	PRO	CARBS	FAT	CALORIES

Evening				
	PRO	CARBS	FAT	CALORIES

Protein Snack				
	PRO	CARBS	FAT	CALORIES

Beverages

Today's Energy Intake
PRO   CARBS   FAT   CALORIES

Daily Activities
ACTIVITY/DURATION

Fitness Exercise
Activity for the purpose of health

/

Activities of Living
Physical movement in the daily routine

/

Extra Mile
Intentional physical activity beyond the necessary: taking stairs, walking vs. transport; standing vs. sitting; etc.

/

Today I was active for:
___Hour ____ Min

Emoji of the Day

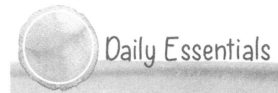 Daily Essentials

Protein First Meals
Protein goal: grams/day

Morning				
	PRO	CARBS	FAT	CALORIES
Midday				
	PRO	CARBS	FAT	CALORIES
Evening				
	PRO	CARBS	FAT	CALORIES
Protein Snack				
	PRO	CARBS	FAT	CALORIES
Beverages				

Today's Energy Intake
PRO   CARBS   FAT   CALORIES

Obstacle Awareness:
Mindful Preparedness

Daily Activities
ACTIVITY/DURATION
Fitness Exercise
Activity for the purpose of health

/

Activities of Living
Physical movement in the daily routine

/

Extra Mile
Intentional physical activity beyond the necessary: taking stairs, walking vs. transport; standing vs. sitting; etc.

/

Today I was active for:

___Hour ____ Min

Emoji of the Day

Daily Essentials

Protein First Meals

Protein goal: _____ grams/day

Morning				
	PRO	CARBS	FAT	CALORIES

Midday				
	PRO	CARBS	FAT	CALORIES

Evening				
	PRO	CARBS	FAT	CALORIES

Protein Snack				
	PRO	CARBS	FAT	CALORIES

Beverages

Today's Energy Intake
PRO   CARBS   FAT   CALORIES

Obstacle Awareness: Mindful Preparedness

Daily Activities
ACTIVITY/DURATION

Fitness Exercise
Activity for the purpose of health

/

Activities of Living
Physical movement in the daily routine

/

Extra Mile
Intentional physical activity beyond the necessary: taking stairs, walking vs. transport; standing vs. sitting; etc.

/

Today I was active for:

_____Hour _____ Min

Emoji of the Day

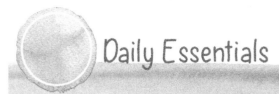

Daily Essentials

Protein First Meals
Protein goal: grams/day

		PRO	CARBS	FAT	CALORIES
Morning					
		PRO	CARBS	FAT	CALORIES
Midday					
		PRO	CARBS	FAT	CALORIES
Evening					
		PRO	CARBS	FAT	CALORIES
Protein Snack					
		PRO	CARBS	FAT	CALORIES
Beverages					

Today's Energy Intake
PRO   CARBS   FAT   CALORIES

Obstacle Awareness:
Mindful Preparedness

Daily Activities
ACTIVITY/DURATION
Fitness Exercise
Activity for the purpose of health

/

Activities of Living
Physical movement in the daily routine

/

Extra Mile
Intentional physical activity beyond the necessary: taking stairs, walking vs. transport; standing vs. sitting; etc.

/

Today I was active for:

____Hour _____ Min

Emoji of the Day

Words & Doodles

New Week: Great Plan

I've got a good feeling about this!
Week of:

Protein First Meals

Monday

Tuesday

Wednesday

Thursday

Friday

Saturday

Sunday

Week 2: Goals

Take a small step to improve your health through diet, fitness, and behavior. Add something; eliminate something; change a habit; try something new.
For each category show: ACTION/REWARD

Diet & Nutrition
/
/

Activities of Living
Physical movement in the daily routine
/
/

Fitness Exercise
Activity for the purpose of health
/
/

Notes:

Grocery List

○   ○   ○   ○

○   ○   ○   ○

○   ○   ○   ○

○   ○   ○   Budget $

○   ○   ○   Actual: $

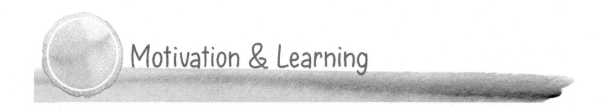

SLIDER FOODS & LIQUID RESTRICTIONS

Slider Foods: To the weight loss surgery patient slider foods are the bane of good intentions often causing dumping syndrome, weight loss plateaus, and eventually weight gain. By definition slider foods are soft simple processed carbohydrates of little or no nutritional value that slide right through the surgical stomach pouch without providing nutrition or satiation. The most commonly consumed slider foods include pretzels, crackers (saltines, graham, Ritz®, etc.) filled cracker snacks such as Ritz Bits®, popcorn, cheese snacks (Cheetos®) or cheese crackers, tortilla chips with salsa, potato chips, sugar-free cookies, cakes, and candy.

The very nature of the surgical gastric pouch is to cause feelings of tightness or restriction when one has eaten enough food. However, when soft simple carbohydrates are eaten this tightness or restriction does not result and one can continue to eat, unmeasured amounts of food without ever feeling uncomfortable. Many patients unknowingly turn to slider foods for this very reason. They do not like the discomfort that results when the pouch is full from eating a measured portion of lean animal or dairy protein, and it is more comfortable to eat the soft slider foods. Slider foods have played a significant role in every case of post-WLS weight regain that I have ever heard about.

Liquid restrictions: After surgical weight loss patients are advised to avoid drinking liquids 30 minutes before meals and 30 minutes after meals. (The time restriction varies from surgeon to surgeon, but most use the 30 minutes before, 30 minutes after restriction. Follow your surgeon's specific directions.) In addition there should be no liquid consumed while eating. Following these liquid restrictions allows the pouch to feel tight sooner and stay tight longer, thus leaving the patient feeling satiated for greater periods of time without experiencing the urge to snack. In addition, the longer food stays in the small gastric pouch the more opportunity the body has to absorb nutrients from that food. The liquid restrictions should be followed when eating all meals and snacks, including protein shakes, protein bars, hearty soups, and solid protein main dishes.

Notes:

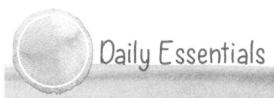 Daily Essentials

Today Is:
S M T W T F S

Protein First Meals

Protein goal: grams/day

Morning				
	PRO	CARBS	FAT	CALORIES
Midday				
	PRO	CARBS	FAT	CALORIES
Evening				
	PRO	CARBS	FAT	CALORIES
Protein Snack				
	PRO	CARBS	FAT	CALORIES

Beverages

Today's Energy Intake

PRO   CARBS   FAT   CALORIES

Obstacle Awareness:
Mindful Preparedness

Daily Activities

ACTIVITY/DURATION

Fitness Exercise
Activity for the purpose of health

/

Activities of Living
Physical movement in the daily routine

/

Extra Mile
*Intentional physical activity beyond the necessary:
taking stairs, walking vs. transport; standing vs.
sitting; etc.*

/

Today I was active for:

___Hour ____ Min

Emoji of the Day

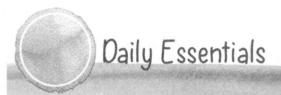

Daily Essentials

Today Is:
S M T W T F S

Protein First Meals

Protein goal: _____ grams/day

Morning				
	PRO	CARBS	FAT	CALORIES
Midday				
	PRO	CARBS	FAT	CALORIES
Evening				
	PRO	CARBS	FAT	CALORIES
Protein Snack				
	PRO	CARBS	FAT	CALORIES
Beverages				

Today's Energy Intake
PRO _____ CARBS _____ FAT _____ CALORIES _____

Obstacle Awareness:
Mindful Preparedness

Daily Activities
ACTIVITY/DURATION
Fitness Exercise
Activity for the purpose of health

/

Activities of Living
Physical movement in the daily routine

/

Extra Mile
Intentional physical activity beyond the necessary: taking stairs, walking vs. transport; standing vs. sitting; etc.

/

Today I was active for:
_____ Hour _____ Min

Emoji of the Day

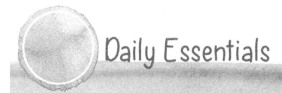

Daily Essentials

Today Is:
S M T W T F S

Protein First Meals
Protein goal: grams/day

Morning				
	PRO	CARBS	FAT	CALORIES
Midday				
	PRO	CARBS	FAT	CALORIES
Evening				
	PRO	CARBS	FAT	CALORIES
Protein Snack				
	PRO	CARBS	FAT	CALORIES

Beverages

Today's Energy Intake
PRO   CARBS   FAT   CALORIES

Obstacle Awareness:
Mindful Preparedness

Daily Activities
ACTIVITY/DURATION
Fitness Exercise
Activity for the purpose of health

/

Activities of Living
Physical movement in the daily routine

/

Extra Mile
Intentional physical activity beyond the necessary: taking stairs, walking vs. transport; standing vs. sitting; etc.

/

Today I was active for:
___Hour ____ Min

Emoji of the Day

Daily Essentials

Today Is:
S M T W T F S

Protein First Meals
Protein goal: grams/day

Morning				
	PRO	CARBS	FAT	CALORIES
Midday				
	PRO	CARBS	FAT	CALORIES
Evening				
	PRO	CARBS	FAT	CALORIES
Protein Snack				
	PRO	CARBS	FAT	CALORIES
Beverages				

Today's Energy Intake
PRO   CARBS   FAT   CALORIES

Obstacle Awareness:
Mindful Preparedness

Daily Activities
ACTIVITY/DURATION
Fitness Exercise
Activity for the purpose of health

/

Activities of Living
Physical movement in the daily routine

/

Extra Mile
Intentional physical activity beyond the necessary: taking stairs, walking vs. transport; standing vs. sitting; etc.

/

Today I was active for:
___Hour ____ Min

Emoji of the Day

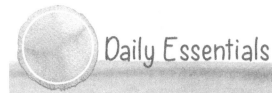

Daily Essentials

Today Is:
S M T W T F S

Protein First Meals

Protein goal: grams/day

Morning				
	PRO	CARBS	FAT	CALORIES
Midday				
	PRO	CARBS	FAT	CALORIES
Evening				
	PRO	CARBS	FAT	CALORIES
Protein Snack				
	PRO	CARBS	FAT	CALORIES
Beverages				

Today's Energy Intake

PRO   CARBS   FAT   CALORIES

| Obstacle Awareness: |
| Mindful Preparedness |

Daily Activities

ACTIVITY/DURATION

Fitness Exercise
Activity for the purpose of health

/

Activities of Living
Physical movement in the daily routine

/

Extra Mile
*Intentional physical activity beyond the necessary:
taking stairs, walking vs. transport; standing vs.
sitting; etc.*

/

Today I was active for:

___Hour ____Min

Emoji of the Day

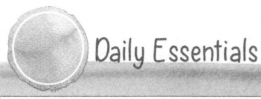 # Daily Essentials

Protein First Meals
Protein goal: grams/day

Morning

PRO	CARBS	FAT	CALORIES

Midday

PRO	CARBS	FAT	CALORIES

Evening

PRO	CARBS	FAT	CALORIES

Protein Snack

PRO	CARBS	FAT	CALORIES

Beverages

Today's Energy Intake
PRO	CARBS	FAT	CALORIES

Obstacle Awareness:
Mindful Preparedness

Daily Activities
ACTIVITY/DURATION
Fitness Exercise
Activity for the purpose of health

/

Activities of Living
Physical movement in the daily routine

/

Extra Mile
Intentional physical activity beyond the necessary: taking stairs, walking vs. transport; standing vs. sitting; etc.

/

Today I was active for:

___Hour ____ Min

Emoji of the Day

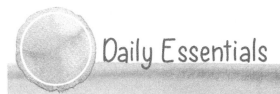 Daily Essentials

Today Is:
S M T W T F S

Protein First Meals
Protein goal: grams/day

Morning				
	PRO	CARBS	FAT	CALORIES
Midday				
	PRO	CARBS	FAT	CALORIES
Evening				
	PRO	CARBS	FAT	CALORIES
Protein Snack				
	PRO	CARBS	FAT	CALORIES
Beverages				

Today's Energy Intake
PRO   CARBS   FAT   CALORIES

Obstacle Awareness:
Mindful Preparedness

Daily Activities
ACTIVITY/DURATION
Fitness Exercise
Activity for the purpose of health

/

Activities of Living
Physical movement in the daily routine

/

Extra Mile
Intentional physical activity beyond the necessary:
taking stairs, walking vs. transport; standing vs.
sitting; etc.

/

Today I was active for:

___Hour ____Min

Emoji of the Day

Words & Doodles

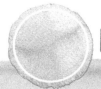

New Week: Great Plan

I've got a good feeling about this!
Week of:

Protein First Meals

Monday	
Tuesday	
Wednesday	
Thursday	
Friday	
Saturday	
Sunday	

Week 3: Goals

Take a small step to improve your health through diet, fitness, and behavior. Add something; eliminate something; change a habit; try something new.
For each category show: ACTION/REWARD

Diet & Nutrition
/
/

Activities of Living
Physical movement in the daily routine
/
/

Fitness Exercise
Activity for the purpose of health
/
/

Notes:

Grocery List

○	○	○	○
○	○	○	○
○	○	○	○
○	○	○	Budget $
○	○	○	Actual: $

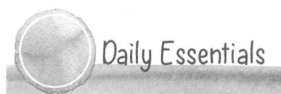

Daily Essentials

Protein First Meals
Protein goal: grams/day

		PRO	CARBS	FAT	CALORIES
Morning					
		PRO	CARBS	FAT	CALORIES
Midday					
		PRO	CARBS	FAT	CALORIES
Evening					
		PRO	CARBS	FAT	CALORIES
Protein Snack					
		PRO	CARBS	FAT	CALORIES
Beverages					

Today's Energy Intake
PRO   CARBS   FAT   CALORIES

---

*Obstacle Awareness:
Mindful Preparedness*

Daily Activities
ACTIVITY/DURATION

Fitness Exercise
Activity for the purpose of health

/

Activities of Living
Physical movement in the daily routine

/

Extra Mile
Intentional physical activity beyond the necessary: taking stairs, walking vs. transport; standing vs. sitting; etc.

/

Today I was active for:

___Hour ____ Min

Emoji of the Day

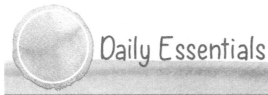 Daily Essentials

Protein First Meals
Protein goal: grams/day

		PRO	CARBS	FAT	CALORIES
Morning					
		PRO	CARBS	FAT	CALORIES
Midday					
		PRO	CARBS	FAT	CALORIES
Evening					
		PRO	CARBS	FAT	CALORIES
Protein Snack					
		PRO	CARBS	FAT	CALORIES
Beverages					

Today's Energy Intake
PRO   CARBS   FAT   CALORIES

*Obstacle Awareness:
Mindful Preparedness*

Daily Activities
ACTIVITY/DURATION
Fitness Exercise
Activity for the purpose of health

/

Activities of Living
Physical movement in the daily routine

/

Extra Mile
Intentional physical activity beyond the necessary: taking stairs, walking vs. transport; standing vs. sitting; etc.

/

Today I was active for:
____Hour _____ Min

Emoji of the Day

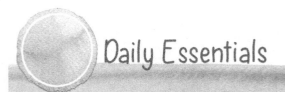 **Daily Essentials**

Protein First Meals

Protein goal: grams/day

Morning

PRO	CARBS	FAT	CALORIES

Midday

PRO	CARBS	FAT	CALORIES

Evening

PRO	CARBS	FAT	CALORIES

Protein Snack

PRO	CARBS	FAT	CALORIES

Beverages

Today's Energy Intake

PRO	CARBS	FAT	CALORIES

---

*Obstacle Awareness:
Mindful Preparedness*

Daily Activities

ACTIVITY/DURATION

Fitness Exercise
Activity for the purpose of health

/

Activities of Living
Physical movement in the daily routine

/

Extra Mile
*Intentional physical activity beyond the necessary:
taking stairs, walking vs. transport; standing vs.
sitting; etc.*

/

Today I was active for:

___Hour ____ Min

Emoji of the Day

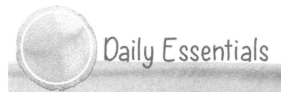 # Daily Essentials

Today Is:
S M T W T F S

Protein First Meals
Protein goal: grams/day

Morning	PRO	CARBS	FAT	CALORIES
Midday	PRO	CARBS	FAT	CALORIES
Evening	PRO	CARBS	FAT	CALORIES
Protein Snack	PRO	CARBS	FAT	CALORIES

Beverages

Today's Energy Intake
PRO   CARBS   FAT   CALORIES

Obstacle Awareness:
Mindful Preparedness

Daily Activities
ACTIVITY/DURATION

Fitness Exercise
Activity for the purpose of health

/

Activities of Living
Physical movement in the daily routine

/

Extra Mile
Intentional physical activity beyond the necessary: taking stairs, walking vs. transport; standing vs. sitting; etc.

/

Today I was active for:

___Hour ____ Min

Emoji of the Day

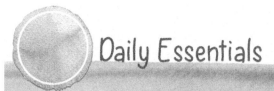 Daily Essentials

Protein First Meals
Protein goal: grams/day

Morning				
	PRO	CARBS	FAT	CALORIES
Midday				
	PRO	CARBS	FAT	CALORIES
Evening				
	PRO	CARBS	FAT	CALORIES
Protein Snack				
	PRO	CARBS	FAT	CALORIES
Beverages				

Today's Energy Intake
PRO   CARBS   FAT   CALORIES

Obstacle Awareness: Mindful Preparedness

Daily Activities
ACTIVITY/DURATION
Fitness Exercise
Activity for the purpose of health

/

Activities of Living
Physical movement in the daily routine

/

Extra Mile
Intentional physical activity beyond the necessary: taking stairs, walking vs. transport; standing vs. sitting; etc.

/

Today I was active for:

____Hour ____ Min

Emoji of the Day

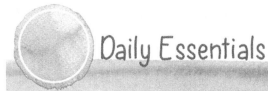

Daily Essentials

Protein First Meals
Protein goal: grams/day

Morning				
	PRO	CARBS	FAT	CALORIES
Midday				
	PRO	CARBS	FAT	CALORIES
Evening				
	PRO	CARBS	FAT	CALORIES
Protein Snack				
	PRO	CARBS	FAT	CALORIES
Beverages				

Today's Energy Intake
PRO   CARBS   FAT   CALORIES

Obstacle Awareness:
Mindful Preparedness

Daily Activities
ACTIVITY/DURATION
Fitness Exercise
Activity for the purpose of health

/

Activities of Living
Physical movement in the daily routine

/

Extra Mile
Intentional physical activity beyond the necessary: taking stairs, walking vs. transport; standing vs. sitting; etc.

/

Today I was active for:

___Hour ____ Min

Emoji of the Day

Daily Essentials

Protein First Meals
Protein goal: grams/day

Morning					
		PRO	CARBS	FAT	CALORIES
Midday					
		PRO	CARBS	FAT	CALORIES
Evening					
		PRO	CARBS	FAT	CALORIES
Protein Snack					
		PRO	CARBS	FAT	CALORIES
Beverages					

Today's Energy Intake
PRO   CARBS   FAT   CALORIES

Obstacle Awareness:
Mindful Preparedness

Daily Activities
ACTIVITY/DURATION

Fitness Exercise
Activity for the purpose of health

/

Activities of Living
Physical movement in the daily routine

/

Extra Mile
Intentional physical activity beyond the necessary: taking stairs, walking vs. transport; standing vs. sitting; etc.

/

Today I was active for:

___Hour ____ Min

Emoji of the Day

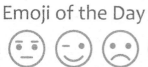

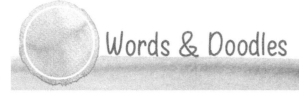

Words & Doodles

New Week: Great Plan

I've got a good feeling about this!
Week of:

Protein First Meals

Monday	
Tuesday	
Wednesday	
Thursday	
Friday	
Saturday	
Sunday	

Week 4: Goals

Take a small step to improve your health through diet, fitness, and behavior. Add something; eliminate something; change a habit; try something new.
For each category show: ACTION/REWARD

Diet & Nutrition
/
/

Activities of Living
Physical movement in the daily routine
/
/

Fitness Exercise
Activity for the purpose of health
/
/

Notes:

Grocery List

○ ○ ○ ○
○ ○ ○ ○
○ ○ ○ ○
○ ○ ○ Budget $
○ ○ ○ Actual: $

Daily Essentials

Today Is:
S M T W T F S

Protein First Meals

Protein goal: grams/day

Morning

PRO	CARBS	FAT	CALORIES

Midday

PRO	CARBS	FAT	CALORIES

Evening

PRO	CARBS	FAT	CALORIES

Protein Snack

PRO	CARBS	FAT	CALORIES

Beverages

Obstacle Awareness:
Mindful Preparedness

Daily Activities

ACTIVITY/DURATION

Fitness Exercise
Activity for the purpose of health

/

Activities of Living
Physical movement in the daily routine

/

Extra Mile
Intentional physical activity beyond the necessary: taking stairs, walking vs. transport; standing vs. sitting; etc.

/

Today I was active for:

____Hour ____ Min

Today's Energy Intake

PRO   CARBS   FAT   CALORIES

Emoji of the Day

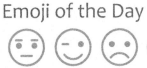

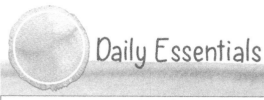

Daily Essentials

Protein First Meals

Protein goal: grams/day

Morning				
	PRO	CARBS	FAT	CALORIES

Midday				
	PRO	CARBS	FAT	CALORIES

Evening				
	PRO	CARBS	FAT	CALORIES

Protein Snack				
	PRO	CARBS	FAT	CALORIES

Beverages

Today's Energy Intake
PRO   CARBS   FAT   CALORIES

Obstacle Awareness:
Mindful Preparedness

Daily Activities
ACTIVITY/DURATION
Fitness Exercise
Activity for the purpose of health

/

Activities of Living
Physical movement in the daily routine

/

Extra Mile
Intentional physical activity beyond the necessary: taking stairs, walking vs. transport; standing vs. sitting; etc.

/

Today I was active for:

___Hour ____ Min

Emoji of the Day

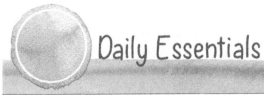 Daily Essentials

Protein First Meals
Protein goal: grams/day

Morning				
	PRO	CARBS	FAT	CALORIES
Midday				
	PRO	CARBS	FAT	CALORIES
Evening				
	PRO	CARBS	FAT	CALORIES
Protein Snack				
	PRO	CARBS	FAT	CALORIES

Beverages

Today's Energy Intake
PRO   CARBS   FAT   CALORIES

Obstacle Awareness:
Mindful Preparedness

Daily Activities
ACTIVITY/DURATION
Fitness Exercise
Activity for the purpose of health

/

Activities of Living
Physical movement in the daily routine

/

Extra Mile
Intentional physical activity beyond the necessary: taking stairs, walking vs. transport; standing vs. sitting; etc.

/

Today I was active for:

____Hour _____ Min

Emoji of the Day

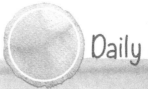

Daily Essentials

Protein First Meals
Protein goal: ___ grams/day

Morning				
	PRO	CARBS	FAT	CALORIES

Midday				
	PRO	CARBS	FAT	CALORIES

Evening				
	PRO	CARBS	FAT	CALORIES

Protein Snack				
	PRO	CARBS	FAT	CALORIES

Beverages

Today's Energy Intake
PRO   CARBS   FAT   CALORIES

Obstacle Awareness:
Mindful Preparedness

Daily Activities
ACTIVITY/DURATION

Fitness Exercise
Activity for the purpose of health

/

Activities of Living
Physical movement in the daily routine

/

Extra Mile
Intentional physical activity beyond the necessary: taking stairs, walking vs. transport; standing vs. sitting; etc.

/

Today I was active for:

___Hour ____ Min

Emoji of the Day

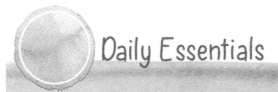

Daily Essentials

Today Is:
S M T W T F S

Protein First Meals

Protein goal: grams/day

Morning				
	PRO	CARBS	FAT	CALORIES

Midday				
	PRO	CARBS	FAT	CALORIES

Evening				
	PRO	CARBS	FAT	CALORIES

Protein Snack				
	PRO	CARBS	FAT	CALORIES

Beverages

Today's Energy Intake
PRO   CARBS   FAT   CALORIES

Obstacle Awareness:
Mindful Preparedness

Daily Activities
ACTIVITY/DURATION
Fitness Exercise
Activity for the purpose of health

/

Activities of Living
Physical movement in the daily routine

/

Extra Mile
Intentional physical activity beyond the necessary: taking stairs, walking vs. transport; standing vs. sitting; etc.

/

Today I was active for:

___Hour _____Min

Emoji of the Day

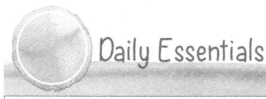

Daily Essentials

Protein First Meals

Protein goal: grams/day

		PRO	CARBS	FAT	CALORIES
Morning					
Midday					
Evening					
Protein Snack					
Beverages					

Today's Energy Intake

PRO   CARBS   FAT   CALORIES

Obstacle Awareness:
Mindful Preparedness

Daily Activities

ACTIVITY/DURATION

Fitness Exercise
Activity for the purpose of health

/

Activities of Living
Physical movement in the daily routine

/

Extra Mile
Intentional physical activity beyond the necessary: taking stairs, walking vs. transport; standing vs. sitting; etc.

/

Today I was active for:

___Hour ____ Min

Emoji of the Day

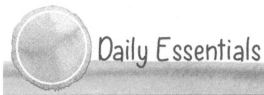

Daily Essentials

Protein First Meals

Protein goal: grams/day

Morning				
	PRO	CARBS	FAT	CALORIES
Midday				
	PRO	CARBS	FAT	CALORIES
Evening				
	PRO	CARBS	FAT	CALORIES
Protein Snack				
	PRO	CARBS	FAT	CALORIES
Beverages				

Today's Energy Intake

PRO   CARBS   FAT   CALORIES

Obstacle Awareness:
Mindful Preparedness

Daily Activities
ACTIVITY/DURATION

Fitness Exercise
Activity for the purpose of health

/

Activities of Living
Physical movement in the daily routine

/

Extra Mile
Intentional physical activity beyond the necessary: taking stairs, walking vs. transport; standing vs. sitting; etc.

/

Today I was active for:

___Hour ____ Min

Emoji of the Day

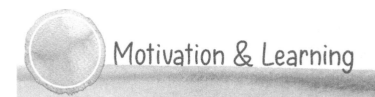

Motivation & Learning

Review of Month 1:

To Do:

Words & Doodles

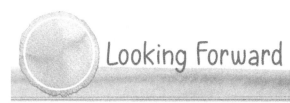

Looking Forward

Month/Year

SUNDAY	MONDAY	TUESDAY	WEDNESDAY	THURSDAY	FRIDAY	SATURDAY

Obstacle Awareness:
Mindful Preparedness

Words & Doodles

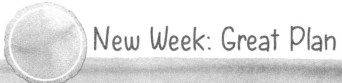

New Week: Great Plan

I've got a good feeling about this!
Week of:

Protein First Meals

Monday	
Tuesday	
Wednesday	
Thursday	
Friday	
Saturday	
Sunday	

Week 5: Goals

Take a small step to improve your health through diet, fitness, and behavior. Add something; eliminate something; change a habit; try something new.
For each category show: ACTION/REWARD

Diet & Nutrition
/
/

Activities of Living
Physical movement in the daily routine
/
/

Fitness Exercise
Activity for the purpose of health
/
/

Notes:

Grocery List

○ ○ ○ ○
○ ○ ○ ○
○ ○ ○ ○
○ ○ ○ Budget $
○ ○ ○ Actual: $

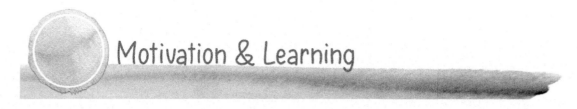

Motivation & Learning

Motivation

One way to motivate yourself is to recognize how gratifying it is to make a goal, identify the specific steps to get there, follow your plan and celebrate the rewards.

Daily Essentials

Protein First Meals
Protein goal: grams/day

Morning				
	PRO	CARBS	FAT	CALORIES
Midday				
	PRO	CARBS	FAT	CALORIES
Evening				
	PRO	CARBS	FAT	CALORIES
Protein Snack				
	PRO	CARBS	FAT	CALORIES
Beverages				

Obstacle Awareness:
Mindful Preparedness

Daily Activities
ACTIVITY/DURATION
Fitness Exercise
Activity for the purpose of health

/

Activities of Living
Physical movement in the daily routine

/

Extra Mile
Intentional physical activity beyond the necessary: taking stairs, walking vs. transport; standing vs. sitting; etc.

/

Today I was active for:
___Hour ____ Min

Today's Energy Intake
PRO   CARBS   FAT   CALORIES

Emoji of the Day

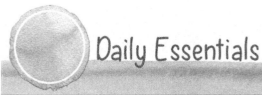

Daily Essentials

Today Is:
S M T W T F S

Protein First Meals

Protein goal: ___ grams/day

Morning	PRO	CARBS	FAT	CALORIES
Midday	PRO	CARBS	FAT	CALORIES
Evening	PRO	CARBS	FAT	CALORIES
Protein Snack	PRO	CARBS	FAT	CALORIES
Beverages				

Today's Energy Intake

PRO   CARBS   FAT   CALORIES

Obstacle Awareness:
Mindful Preparedness

Daily Activities

ACTIVITY/DURATION

Fitness Exercise
Activity for the purpose of health

/

Activities of Living
Physical movement in the daily routine

/

Extra Mile
Intentional physical activity beyond the necessary: taking stairs, walking vs. transport; standing vs. sitting; etc.

/

Today I was active for:

___Hour ____ Min

Emoji of the Day

Daily Essentials

Today Is:
S M T W T F S

Protein First Meals

Protein goal: grams/day

Morning	PRO	CARBS	FAT	CALORIES
Midday	PRO	CARBS	FAT	CALORIES
Evening	PRO	CARBS	FAT	CALORIES
Protein Snack	PRO	CARBS	FAT	CALORIES

Beverages

Today's Energy Intake
PRO   CARBS   FAT   CALORIES

Obstacle Awareness:
Mindful Preparedness

Daily Activities
ACTIVITY/DURATION

Fitness Exercise
Activity for the purpose of health

/

Activities of Living
Physical movement in the daily routine

/

Extra Mile
Intentional physical activity beyond the necessary: taking stairs, walking vs. transport; standing vs. sitting; etc.

/

Today I was active for:

___Hour ____ Min

Emoji of the Day

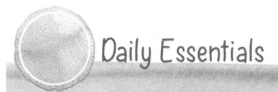 Daily Essentials

Today Is:
S M T W T F S

Protein First Meals
Protein goal: grams/day

Morning				
	PRO	CARBS	FAT	CALORIES
Midday				
	PRO	CARBS	FAT	CALORIES
Evening				
	PRO	CARBS	FAT	CALORIES
Protein Snack				
	PRO	CARBS	FAT	CALORIES

Beverages

Obstacle Awareness:
Mindful Preparedness

Daily Activities
ACTIVITY/DURATION
Fitness Exercise
Activity for the purpose of health

/

Activities of Living
Physical movement in the daily routine

/

Extra Mile
Intentional physical activity beyond the necessary: taking stairs, walking vs. transport; standing vs. sitting; etc.

/

Today I was active for:
___Hour ____ Min

Today's Energy Intake
PRO   CARBS   FAT   CALORIES

Emoji of the Day

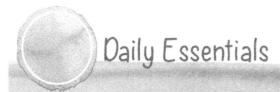 Daily Essentials

Today Is:
S M T W T F S

Protein First Meals

Protein goal: grams/day

Morning				
	PRO	CARBS	FAT	CALORIES

Midday				
	PRO	CARBS	FAT	CALORIES

Evening				
	PRO	CARBS	FAT	CALORIES

Protein Snack				
	PRO	CARBS	FAT	CALORIES

Beverages

Obstacle Awareness:
Mindful Preparedness

Daily Activities

ACTIVITY/DURATION

Fitness Exercise
Activity for the purpose of health

/

Activities of Living
Physical movement in the daily routine

/

Extra Mile
Intentional physical activity beyond the necessary:
taking stairs, walking vs. transport; standing vs.
sitting; etc.

/

Today I was active for:

___Hour ____ Min

Today's Energy Intake

PRO   CARBS   FAT   CALORIES

Emoji of the Day

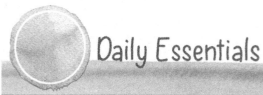 Daily Essentials

Protein First Meals
Protein goal: grams/day

Morning		
	PRO CARBS FAT CALORIES	
Midday		
	PRO CARBS FAT CALORIES	
Evening		
	PRO CARBS FAT CALORIES	
Protein Snack		
	PRO CARBS FAT CALORIES	
Beverages		

Today's Energy Intake
PRO   CARBS   FAT   CALORIES

Obstacle Awareness:
Mindful Preparedness

Daily Activities
ACTIVITY/DURATION
Fitness Exercise
Activity for the purpose of health

/

Activities of Living
Physical movement in the daily routine

/

Extra Mile
Intentional physical activity beyond the necessary:
taking stairs, walking vs. transport; standing vs.
sitting; etc.

/

Today I was active for:

___Hour ____ Min

Emoji of the Day

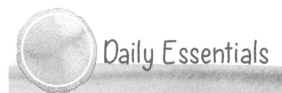

Daily Essentials

Protein First Meals
Protein goal: grams/day

	Morning			
Morning	PRO	CARBS	FAT	CALORIES
Midday	PRO	CARBS	FAT	CALORIES
Evening	PRO	CARBS	FAT	CALORIES
Protein Snack	PRO	CARBS	FAT	CALORIES

Beverages

Today's Energy Intake
PRO   CARBS   FAT   CALORIES

Obstacle Awareness:
Mindful Preparedness

Daily Activities
ACTIVITY/DURATION

Fitness Exercise
Activity for the purpose of health

/

Activities of Living
Physical movement in the daily routine

/

Extra Mile
Intentional physical activity beyond the necessary:
taking stairs, walking vs. transport; standing vs.
sitting; etc.

/

Today I was active for:

____Hour _____ Min

Emoji of the Day

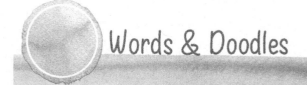

Words & Doodles

New Week: Great Plan

I've got a good feeling about this!
Week of:

Protein First Meals

Monday	
Tuesday	
Wednesday	
Thursday	
Friday	
Saturday	
Sunday	

Week 6: Goals

Take a small step to improve your health through diet, fitness, and behavior. Add something; eliminate something; change a habit; try something new.
For each category show: ACTION/REWARD

Diet & Nutrition

/

/

Activities of Living

Physical movement in the daily routine

/

/

Fitness Exercise

Activity for the purpose of health

/

/

Notes:

Grocery List

○ ○ ○ ○
○ ○ ○ ○
○ ○ ○ ○
○ ○ ○ Budget $
○ ○ ○ Actual: $

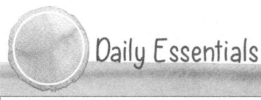

Daily Essentials

Protein First Meals
Protein goal: grams/day

Morning				
	PRO	CARBS	FAT	CALORIES
Midday				
	PRO	CARBS	FAT	CALORIES
Evening				
	PRO	CARBS	FAT	CALORIES
Protein Snack				
	PRO	CARBS	FAT	CALORIES

Beverages

Today's Energy Intake
PRO   CARBS   FAT   CALORIES

Obstacle Awareness:
Mindful Preparedness

Daily Activities
ACTIVITY/DURATION
Fitness Exercise
Activity for the purpose of health

/

Activities of Living
Physical movement in the daily routine

/

Extra Mile
Intentional physical activity beyond the necessary: taking stairs, walking vs. transport; standing vs. sitting; etc.

/

Today I was active for:
____Hour _____ Min

Emoji of the Day
🙂 😐 😉 ☹️ ⚪

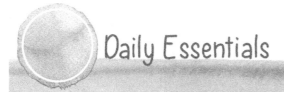 Daily Essentials

Today Is:
S M T W T F S

Protein First Meals
Protein goal: grams/day

Morning	
	PRO CARBS FAT CALORIES
Midday	
	PRO CARBS FAT CALORIES
Evening	
	PRO CARBS FAT CALORIES
Protein Snack	
	PRO CARBS FAT CALORIES
Beverages	

Today's Energy Intake
PRO   CARBS   FAT   CALORIES

Obstacle Awareness:
Mindful Preparedness

Daily Activities
ACTIVITY/DURATION
Fitness Exercise
Activity for the purpose of health

/

Activities of Living
Physical movement in the daily routine

/

Extra Mile
Intentional physical activity beyond the necessary: taking stairs, walking vs. transport; standing vs. sitting; etc.

/

Today I was active for:
____Hour _____ Min

Emoji of the Day

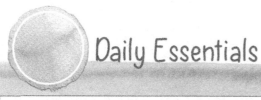

Daily Essentials

Protein First Meals
Protein goal: grams/day

Morning				
	PRO	CARBS	FAT	CALORIES
Midday				
	PRO	CARBS	FAT	CALORIES
Evening				
	PRO	CARBS	FAT	CALORIES
Protein Snack				
	PRO	CARBS	FAT	CALORIES

Beverages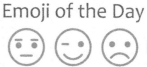

Today's Energy Intake
PRO   CARBS   FAT   CALORIES

Obstacle Awareness:
Mindful Preparedness

Daily Activities
ACTIVITY/DURATION

Fitness Exercise
Activity for the purpose of health

/

Activities of Living
Physical movement in the daily routine

/

Extra Mile
Intentional physical activity beyond the necessary: taking stairs, walking vs. transport; standing vs. sitting; etc.

/

Today I was active for:

___Hour ____ Min

Emoji of the Day

☺ 😐 😉 ☹ ◯

Daily Essentials

Protein First Meals

Protein goal: grams/day

Morning				
	PRO	CARBS	FAT	CALORIES

Midday				
	PRO	CARBS	FAT	CALORIES

Evening				
	PRO	CARBS	FAT	CALORIES

Protein Snack				
	PRO	CARBS	FAT	CALORIES

Beverages

Obstacle Awareness: Mindful Preparedness

Daily Activities
ACTIVITY/DURATION

Fitness Exercise
Activity for the purpose of health

/

Activities of Living
Physical movement in the daily routine

/

Extra Mile
Intentional physical activity beyond the necessary: taking stairs, walking vs. transport; standing vs. sitting; etc.

/

Today I was active for:

____Hour _____ Min

Today's Energy Intake

PRO   CARBS   FAT   CALORIES

Emoji of the Day

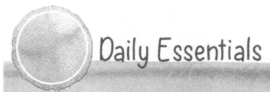

Daily Essentials

Protein First Meals
Protein goal: grams/day

Morning

PRO	CARBS	FAT	CALORIES

Midday

PRO	CARBS	FAT	CALORIES

Evening

PRO	CARBS	FAT	CALORIES

Protein Snack

PRO	CARBS	FAT	CALORIES

Beverages

Today's Energy Intake

PRO	CARBS	FAT	CALORIES

Obstacle Awareness:
Mindful Preparedness

Daily Activities
ACTIVITY/DURATION

Fitness Exercise
Activity for the purpose of health

/

Activities of Living
Physical movement in the daily routine

/

Extra Mile
Intentional physical activity beyond the necessary: taking stairs, walking vs. transport; standing vs. sitting; etc.

/

Today I was active for:

____Hour _____ Min

Emoji of the Day

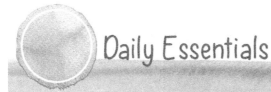 Daily Essentials

Protein First Meals
Protein goal: grams/day

Morning				
	PRO	CARBS	FAT	CALORIES

Midday				
	PRO	CARBS	FAT	CALORIES

Evening				
	PRO	CARBS	FAT	CALORIES

Protein Snack				
	PRO	CARBS	FAT	CALORIES

Beverages

Today's Energy Intake
PRO   CARBS   FAT   CALORIES

Obstacle Awareness:
Mindful Preparedness

Daily Activities
ACTIVITY/DURATION
Fitness Exercise
Activity for the purpose of health

/

Activities of Living
Physical movement in the daily routine

/

Extra Mile
Intentional physical activity beyond the necessary: taking stairs, walking vs. transport; standing vs. sitting; etc.

/

Today I was active for:

____Hour _____ Min

Emoji of the Day
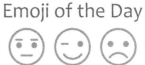

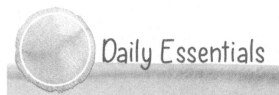

Daily Essentials

Today Is:
S M T W T F S

Protein First Meals
Protein goal: _____ grams/day

Morning					
		PRO	CARBS	FAT	CALORIES
Midday					
		PRO	CARBS	FAT	CALORIES
Evening					
		PRO	CARBS	FAT	CALORIES
Protein Snack					
		PRO	CARBS	FAT	CALORIES
Beverages					

Today's Energy Intake
PRO   CARBS   FAT   CALORIES

Obstacle Awareness:
Mindful Preparedness

Daily Activities
ACTIVITY/DURATION

Fitness Exercise
Activity for the purpose of health

/

Activities of Living
Physical movement in the daily routine

/

Extra Mile
Intentional physical activity beyond the necessary: taking stairs, walking vs. transport; standing vs. sitting; etc.

/

Today I was active for:

_____ Hour _____ Min

Emoji of the Day

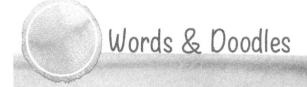

Words & Doodles

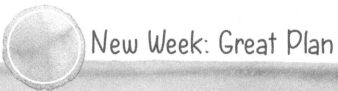

New Week: Great Plan

I've got a good feeling about this!
Week of:

Protein First Meals

Monday	
Tuesday	
Wednesday	
Thursday	
Friday	
Saturday	
Sunday	

Week 7: Goals

Take a small step to improve your health through diet, fitness, and behavior. Add something; eliminate something; change a habit; try something new.
For each category show: ACTION/REWARD

Diet & Nutrition
/
/

Activities of Living
Physical movement in the daily routine
/
/

Fitness Exercise
Activity for the purpose of health
/
/

Notes:

Grocery List

○   ○   ○   ○
○   ○   ○   ○
○   ○   ○   ○
○   ○   ○   Budget $
○   ○   ○   Actual: $

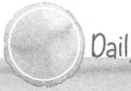

Daily Essentials

Protein First Meals

Protein goal: grams/day

Morning	
	PRO CARBS FAT CALORIES
Midday	
	PRO CARBS FAT CALORIES
Evening	
	PRO CARBS FAT CALORIES
Protein Snack	
	PRO CARBS FAT CALORIES
Beverages	

Today's Energy Intake
PRO   CARBS   FAT   CALORIES

Obstacle Awareness:
Mindful Preparedness

Daily Activities
ACTIVITY/DURATION

Fitness Exercise
Activity for the purpose of health

/

Activities of Living
Physical movement in the daily routine

/

Extra Mile
Intentional physical activity beyond the necessary:
taking stairs, walking vs. transport; standing vs.
sitting; etc.

/

Today I was active for:

___Hour ____Min

Emoji of the Day

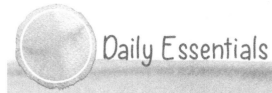

Daily Essentials

Protein First Meals

Protein goal: grams/day

Morning	
	PRO CARBS FAT CALORIES
Midday	
	PRO CARBS FAT CALORIES
Evening	
	PRO CARBS FAT CALORIES
Protein Snack	
	PRO CARBS FAT CALORIES
Beverages	

Today's Energy Intake

PRO   CARBS   FAT   CALORIES

Obstacle Awareness:
Mindful Preparedness

Daily Activities

ACTIVITY/DURATION

Fitness Exercise
Activity for the purpose of health

/

Activities of Living
Physical movement in the daily routine

/

Extra Mile
Intentional physical activity beyond the necessary: taking stairs, walking vs. transport; standing vs. sitting; etc.

/

Today I was active for:

___Hour ____ Min

Emoji of the Day

☺ 😐 🙂 ☹ ◯

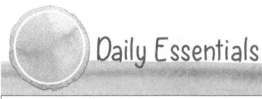 Daily Essentials

Protein First Meals
Protein goal: grams/day

		PRO	CARBS	FAT	CALORIES
Morning					
		PRO	CARBS	FAT	CALORIES
Midday					
		PRO	CARBS	FAT	CALORIES
Evening					
		PRO	CARBS	FAT	CALORIES
Protein Snack					
		PRO	CARBS	FAT	CALORIES
Beverages					

Today's Energy Intake
PRO   CARBS   FAT   CALORIES

Obstacle Awareness:
Mindful Preparedness

Daily Activities
ACTIVITY/DURATION
Fitness Exercise
Activity for the purpose of health

/

Activities of Living
Physical movement in the daily routine

/

Extra Mile
*Intentional physical activity beyond the necessary:
taking stairs, walking vs. transport; standing vs.
sitting; etc.*

/

Today I was active for:
___Hour ____ Min

Emoji of the Day

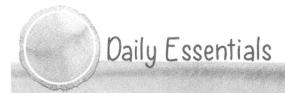

Daily Essentials

Today Is:
S M T W T F S

Protein First Meals

Protein goal: grams/day

Morning				
	PRO	CARBS	FAT	CALORIES
Midday				
	PRO	CARBS	FAT	CALORIES
Evening				
	PRO	CARBS	FAT	CALORIES
Protein Snack				
	PRO	CARBS	FAT	CALORIES
Beverages				

Today's Energy Intake

PRO   CARBS   FAT   CALORIES

Obstacle Awareness:
Mindful Preparedness

Daily Activities

ACTIVITY/DURATION

Fitness Exercise
Activity for the purpose of health

/

Activities of Living
Physical movement in the daily routine

/

Extra Mile
Intentional physical activity beyond the necessary:
taking stairs, walking vs. transport; standing vs.
sitting; etc.

/

Today I was active for:

___Hour ____ Min

Emoji of the Day

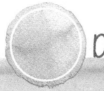

Daily Essentials

Protein First Meals
Protein goal: grams/day

Morning				
	PRO	CARBS	FAT	CALORIES
Midday				
	PRO	CARBS	FAT	CALORIES
Evening				
	PRO	CARBS	FAT	CALORIES
Protein Snack				
	PRO	CARBS	FAT	CALORIES
Beverages				

Today's Energy Intake
PRO   CARBS   FAT   CALORIES

Obstacle Awareness:
Mindful Preparedness

Daily Activities
ACTIVITY/DURATION

Fitness Exercise
Activity for the purpose of health

/

Activities of Living
Physical movement in the daily routine

/

Extra Mile
*Intentional physical activity beyond the necessary:
taking stairs, walking vs. transport; standing vs.
sitting; etc.*

/

Today I was active for:

___Hour ____ Min

Emoji of the Day

Daily Essentials

Protein First Meals

Protein goal: grams/day

Morning	PRO	CARBS	FAT	CALORIES
Midday	PRO	CARBS	FAT	CALORIES
Evening	PRO	CARBS	FAT	CALORIES
Protein Snack	PRO	CARBS	FAT	CALORIES
Beverages				

Obstacle Awareness:
Mindful Preparedness

Daily Activities
ACTIVITY/DURATION

Fitness Exercise
Activity for the purpose of health

/

Activities of Living
Physical movement in the daily routine

/

Extra Mile
Intentional physical activity beyond the necessary: taking stairs, walking vs. transport; standing vs. sitting; etc.

/

Today I was active for:

___Hour ____ Min

Today's Energy Intake

PRO   CARBS   FAT   CALORIES

Emoji of the Day

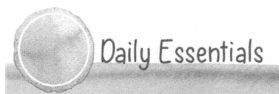

Daily Essentials

Today Is:
S M T W T F S

Protein First Meals
Protein goal: grams/day

		PRO	CARBS	FAT	CALORIES
Morning					
		PRO	CARBS	FAT	CALORIES
Midday					
		PRO	CARBS	FAT	CALORIES
Evening					
		PRO	CARBS	FAT	CALORIES
Protein Snack					
		PRO	CARBS	FAT	CALORIES
Beverages					

Today's Energy Intake
PRO   CARBS   FAT   CALORIES

Obstacle Awareness:
Mindful Preparedness

Daily Activities
ACTIVITY/DURATION

Fitness Exercise
Activity for the purpose of health

/

Activities of Living
Physical movement in the daily routine

/

Extra Mile
Intentional physical activity beyond the necessary:
taking stairs, walking vs. transport; standing vs.
sitting; etc.

/

Today I was active for:

____Hour ____ Min

Emoji of the Day

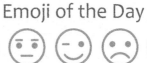

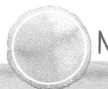

New Week: Great Plan

I've got a good feeling about this!
Week of:

Protein First Meals

Monday	
Tuesday	
Wednesday	
Thursday	
Friday	
Saturday	
Sunday	

Week 8: Goals

Take a small step to improve your health through diet, fitness, and behavior. Add something; eliminate something; change a habit; try something new.
For each category show: ACTION/REWARD

Diet & Nutrition
/
/

Activities of Living
Physical movement in the daily routine
/
/

Fitness Exercise
Activity for the purpose of health
/
/

Notes:

Grocery List

○   ○   ○   ○

○   ○   ○   ○

○   ○   ○   ○

○   ○   ○   Budget $

○   ○   ○   Actual: $

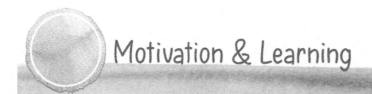

Perfection

We do not have to manage our plate with an all-or-nothing mindset.
This has never worked for keeping our obesity under control.
We must find the happy place between perfection and imperfection.

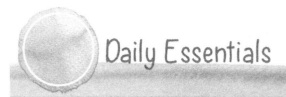
Daily Essentials

Today Is:
S M T W T F S

Protein First Meals

Protein goal: grams/day

Morning				
	PRO	CARBS	FAT	CALORIES
Midday				
	PRO	CARBS	FAT	CALORIES
Evening				
	PRO	CARBS	FAT	CALORIES
Protein Snack				
	PRO	CARBS	FAT	CALORIES

Beverages

Today's Energy Intake
PRO   CARBS   FAT   CALORIES

Obstacle Awareness:
Mindful Preparedness

Daily Activities
ACTIVITY/DURATION
Fitness Exercise
Activity for the purpose of health

/

Activities of Living
Physical movement in the daily routine

/

Extra Mile
Intentional physical activity beyond the necessary: taking stairs, walking vs. transport; standing vs. sitting; etc.

/

Today I was active for:

___Hour ____ Min

Emoji of the Day

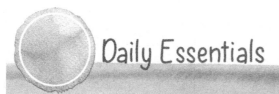
Daily Essentials

Protein First Meals
Protein goal: grams/day

		PRO	CARBS	FAT	CALORIES
Morning					
		PRO	CARBS	FAT	CALORIES
Midday					
		PRO	CARBS	FAT	CALORIES
Evening					
		PRO	CARBS	FAT	CALORIES
Protein Snack					
		PRO	CARBS	FAT	CALORIES
Beverages					

Today's Energy Intake
PRO   CARBS   FAT   CALORIES

Obstacle Awareness:
Mindful Preparedness

Daily Activities
ACTIVITY/DURATION
Fitness Exercise
Activity for the purpose of health

/

Activities of Living
Physical movement in the daily routine

/

Extra Mile
Intentional physical activity beyond the necessary: taking stairs, walking vs. transport; standing vs. sitting; etc.

/

Today I was active for:

____Hour ـ____ Min

Emoji of the Day

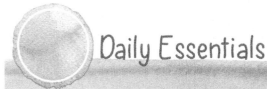

Daily Essentials

Today Is:
S M T W T F S

Protein First Meals
Protein goal: grams/day

		PRO	CARBS	FAT	CALORIES
Morning					
		PRO	CARBS	FAT	CALORIES
Midday					
		PRO	CARBS	FAT	CALORIES
Evening					
		PRO	CARBS	FAT	CALORIES
Protein Snack					
		PRO	CARBS	FAT	CALORIES
Beverages					

Today's Energy Intake
PRO   CARBS   FAT   CALORIES

Obstacle Awareness:
Mindful Preparedness

Daily Activities
ACTIVITY/DURATION
Fitness Exercise
Activity for the purpose of health

/

Activities of Living
Physical movement in the daily routine

/

Extra Mile
Intentional physical activity beyond the necessary: taking stairs, walking vs. transport; standing vs. sitting; etc.

/

Today I was active for:

____Hour ____ Min

Emoji of the Day

Daily Essentials

Today Is:
S M T W T F S

Protein First Meals

Protein goal: grams/day

Morning				
	PRO	CARBS	FAT	CALORIES

Midday				
	PRO	CARBS	FAT	CALORIES

Evening				
	PRO	CARBS	FAT	CALORIES

Protein Snack				
	PRO	CARBS	FAT	CALORIES

Beverages

Today's Energy Intake

PRO   CARBS   FAT   CALORIES

Obstacle Awareness:
Mindful Preparedness

Daily Activities
ACTIVITY/DURATION

Fitness Exercise
Activity for the purpose of health

/

Activities of Living
Physical movement in the daily routine

/

Extra Mile
Intentional physical activity beyond the necessary: taking stairs, walking vs. transport; standing vs. sitting; etc.

/

Today I was active for:

___Hour ____ Min

Emoji of the Day

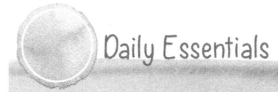

Daily Essentials

Protein First Meals

Protein goal: grams/day

Morning	PRO	CARBS	FAT	CALORIES
Midday	PRO	CARBS	FAT	CALORIES
Evening	PRO	CARBS	FAT	CALORIES
Protein Snack	PRO	CARBS	FAT	CALORIES
Beverages				

Today's Energy Intake

PRO   CARBS   FAT   CALORIES

Obstacle Awareness: Mindful Preparedness

Daily Activities
ACTIVITY/DURATION

Fitness Exercise
Activity for the purpose of health

/

Activities of Living
Physical movement in the daily routine

/

Extra Mile
Intentional physical activity beyond the necessary: taking stairs, walking vs. transport; standing vs. sitting; etc.

/

Today I was active for:

____Hour ____ Min

Emoji of the Day

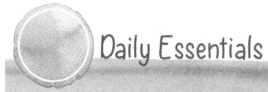

Daily Essentials

Protein First Meals

Protein goal: grams/day

Morning				
	PRO	CARBS	FAT	CALORIES

Midday				
	PRO	CARBS	FAT	CALORIES

Evening				
	PRO	CARBS	FAT	CALORIES

Protein Snack				
	PRO	CARBS	FAT	CALORIES

Beverages

Today's Energy Intake
PRO   CARBS   FAT   CALORIES

Obstacle Awareness:
Mindful Preparedness

Daily Activities
ACTIVITY/DURATION

Fitness Exercise
Activity for the purpose of health

/

Activities of Living
Physical movement in the daily routine

/

Extra Mile
Intentional physical activity beyond the necessary: taking stairs, walking vs. transport; standing vs. sitting; etc.

/

Today I was active for:

___Hour ____Min

Emoji of the Day

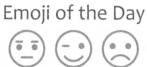

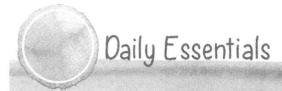

Daily Essentials

Today Is:
S M T W T F S

Protein First Meals
Protein goal: grams/day

		PRO	CARBS	FAT	CALORIES
Morning					
		PRO	CARBS	FAT	CALORIES
Midday					
		PRO	CARBS	FAT	CALORIES
Evening					
		PRO	CARBS	FAT	CALORIES
Protein Snack					
		PRO	CARBS	FAT	CALORIES
Beverages					

Today's Energy Intake
PRO   CARBS   FAT   CALORIES

Obstacle Awareness:
Mindful Preparedness

Daily Activities
ACTIVITY/DURATION
Fitness Exercise
Activity for the purpose of health

/

Activities of Living
Physical movement in the daily routine

/

Extra Mile
Intentional physical activity beyond the necessary: taking stairs, walking vs. transport; standing vs. sitting; etc.

/

Today I was active for:

___Hour ____ Min

Emoji of the Day

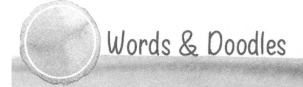

Words & Doodles

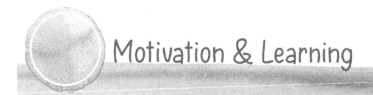

Motivation & Learning

Review of Month 2:

Words & Doodles

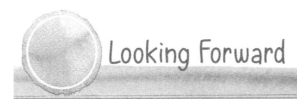

Looking Forward

Month/Year

SUNDAY	MONDAY	TUESDAY	WEDNESDAY	THURSDAY	FRIDAY	SATURDAY

Obstacle Awareness:
Mindful Preparedness

Words & Doodles

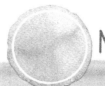

New Week: Great Plan

Protein First Meals

Monday	
Tuesday	
Wednesday	
Thursday	
Friday	
Saturday	
Sunday	

Week 9: Goals

Take a small step to improve your health through diet, fitness, and behavior. Add something; eliminate something; change a habit; try something new.
For each category show: ACTION/REWARD

Diet & Nutrition

/

/

Activities of Living

Physical movement in the daily routine

/

/

Fitness Exercise

Activity for the purpose of health

/

/

Notes:

Grocery List

○ ○ ○ ○
○ ○ ○ ○
○ ○ ○ ○
○ ○ ○ Budget $
○ ○ ○ Actual: $

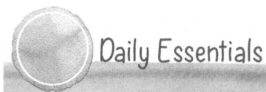 Daily Essentials

Today Is:
S M T W T F S

Protein First Meals
Protein goal: grams/day

		PRO	CARBS	FAT	CALORIES
Morning					
		PRO	CARBS	FAT	CALORIES
Midday					
		PRO	CARBS	FAT	CALORIES
Evening					
		PRO	CARBS	FAT	CALORIES
Protein Snack					
		PRO	CARBS	FAT	CALORIES
Beverages					

Obstacle Awareness:
Mindful Preparedness

Daily Activities
ACTIVITY/DURATION
Fitness Exercise
Activity for the purpose of health

/

Activities of Living
Physical movement in the daily routine

/

Extra Mile
Intentional physical activity beyond the necessary:
taking stairs, walking vs. transport; standing vs.
sitting; etc.

/

Today I was active for:

___Hour ____ Min

Today's Energy Intake
PRO   CARBS   FAT   CALORIES

Emoji of the Day

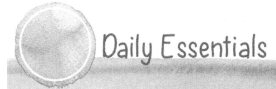

Daily Essentials

Protein First Meals
Protein goal: grams/day

Morning	PRO	CARBS	FAT	CALORIES
Midday	PRO	CARBS	FAT	CALORIES
Evening	PRO	CARBS	FAT	CALORIES
Protein Snack	PRO	CARBS	FAT	CALORIES

Beverages

Today's Energy Intake
PRO   CARBS   FAT   CALORIES

Obstacle Awareness:
Mindful Preparedness

Daily Activities

ACTIVITY/DURATION

Fitness Exercise
Activity for the purpose of health

/

Activities of Living
Physical movement in the daily routine

/

Extra Mile
Intentional physical activity beyond the necessary: taking stairs, walking vs. transport; standing vs. sitting; etc.

/

Today I was active for:

____Hour ____Min

Emoji of the Day

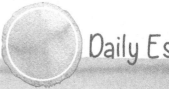 Daily Essentials

Protein First Meals

Protein goal: grams/day

Morning

| PRO | CARBS | FAT | CALORIES |

Midday

| PRO | CARBS | FAT | CALORIES |

Evening

| PRO | CARBS | FAT | CALORIES |

Protein Snack

| PRO | CARBS | FAT | CALORIES |

Beverages

Today's Energy Intake

| PRO | CARBS | FAT | CALORIES |

Obstacle Awareness:
Mindful Preparedness

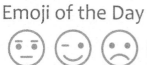

Daily Activities
ACTIVITY/DURATION

Fitness Exercise
Activity for the purpose of health

/

Activities of Living
Physical movement in the daily routine

/

Extra Mile
Intentional physical activity beyond the necessary: taking stairs, walking vs. transport; standing vs. sitting; etc.

/

Today I was active for:

___Hour ____ Min

Emoji of the Day

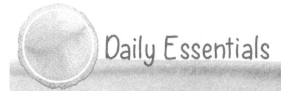

Daily Essentials

Protein First Meals

Protein goal: grams/day

Morning				
	PRO	CARBS	FAT	CALORIES
Midday				
	PRO	CARBS	FAT	CALORIES
Evening				
	PRO	CARBS	FAT	CALORIES
Protein Snack				
	PRO	CARBS	FAT	CALORIES

Beverages

Today's Energy Intake

PRO   CARBS   FAT   CALORIES

Obstacle Awareness: Mindful Preparedness

Daily Activities
ACTIVITY/DURATION

Fitness Exercise
Activity for the purpose of health

/

Activities of Living
Physical movement in the daily routine

/

Extra Mile
Intentional physical activity beyond the necessary: taking stairs, walking vs. transport; standing vs. sitting; etc.

/

Today I was active for:

___Hour ____ Min

Emoji of the Day

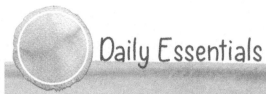 Daily Essentials

Today Is:
S M T W T F S

Protein First Meals
Protein goal: grams/day

Morning	PRO	CARBS	FAT	CALORIES
Midday	PRO	CARBS	FAT	CALORIES
Evening	PRO	CARBS	FAT	CALORIES
Protein Snack	PRO	CARBS	FAT	CALORIES

Beverages

Today's Energy Intake
PRO   CARBS   FAT   CALORIES

Obstacle Awareness:
Mindful Preparedness

Daily Activities
ACTIVITY/DURATION
Fitness Exercise
Activity for the purpose of health

/

Activities of Living
Physical movement in the daily routine

/

Extra Mile
Intentional physical activity beyond the necessary: taking stairs, walking vs. transport; standing vs. sitting; etc.

/

Today I was active for:
___Hour ____ Min

Emoji of the Day

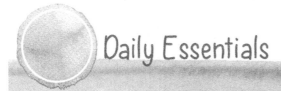

Daily Essentials

Protein First Meals

Protein goal: grams/day

Morning				
	PRO	CARBS	FAT	CALORIES
Midday				
	PRO	CARBS	FAT	CALORIES
Evening				
	PRO	CARBS	FAT	CALORIES
Protein Snack				
	PRO	CARBS	FAT	CALORIES

Beverages

Today's Energy Intake

PRO   CARBS   FAT   CALORIES

Obstacle Awareness:
Mindful Preparedness

Daily Activities

ACTIVITY/DURATION

Fitness Exercise
Activity for the purpose of health

/

Activities of Living
Physical movement in the daily routine

/

Extra Mile
Intentional physical activity beyond the necessary: taking stairs, walking vs. transport; standing vs. sitting; etc.

/

Today I was active for:

___Hour ____ Min

Emoji of the Day

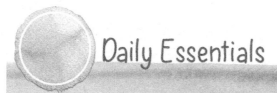

Daily Essentials

Protein First Meals

Protein goal: grams/day

		PRO	CARBS	FAT	CALORIES
Morning					
Midday					
Evening					
Protein Snack					

Beverages

Obstacle Awareness:
Mindful Preparedness

Daily Activities

ACTIVITY/DURATION

Fitness Exercise
Activity for the purpose of health

/

Activities of Living
Physical movement in the daily routine

/

Extra Mile
Intentional physical activity beyond the necessary: taking stairs, walking vs. transport; standing vs. sitting; etc.

/

Today I was active for:

____ Hour _____ Min

Today's Energy Intake
PRO   CARBS   FAT   CALORIES

Emoji of the Day

☺ 😐 🙂 ☹ ◯

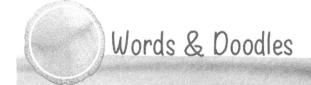

Words & Doodles

New Week: Great Plan

Protein First Meals

Monday	
Tuesday	
Wednesday	
Thursday	
Friday	
Saturday	
Sunday	

Week 10: Goals

Take a small step to improve your health through diet, fitness, and behavior. Add something; eliminate something; change a habit; try something new.
For each category show: ACTION/REWARD

Diet & Nutrition
/
/

Activities of Living
Physical movement in the daily routine
/
/

Fitness Exercise
Activity for the purpose of health
/
/

Notes:

Grocery List

○
○
○
○
○

○
○
○
○
○

○
○
○
○
○

○
○
○

Budget $
Actual: $

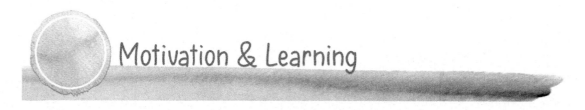

Competition

Losing weight is a matter of health: it is not a competitive sport. Contrary to popular culture, weight loss is not a contest. Weight loss is a lifesaving initiative owned by the one acting to improve their condition. This is your journey: enjoy it at your pace.

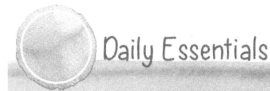

Daily Essentials

Today Is:
S M T W T F S

Protein First Meals
Protein goal: grams/day

Morning				
	PRO	CARBS	FAT	CALORIES
Midday				
	PRO	CARBS	FAT	CALORIES
Evening				
	PRO	CARBS	FAT	CALORIES
Protein Snack				
	PRO	CARBS	FAT	CALORIES
Beverages				

Today's Energy Intake
PRO   CARBS   FAT   CALORIES

Obstacle Awareness:
Mindful Preparedness

Daily Activities
ACTIVITY/DURATION

Fitness Exercise
Activity for the purpose of health

/

Activities of Living
Physical movement in the daily routine

/

Extra Mile
Intentional physical activity beyond the necessary: taking stairs, walking vs. transport; standing vs. sitting; etc.

/

Today I was active for:

___Hour _____ Min

Emoji of the Day

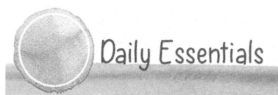 Daily Essentials

Protein First Meals

Protein goal: grams/day

		PRO	CARBS	FAT	CALORIES
Morning					
		PRO	CARBS	FAT	CALORIES
Midday					
		PRO	CARBS	FAT	CALORIES
Evening					
		PRO	CARBS	FAT	CALORIES
Protein Snack					
		PRO	CARBS	FAT	CALORIES
Beverages					

Today's Energy Intake

PRO	CARBS	FAT	CALORIES

Obstacle Awareness:
Mindful Preparedness

Daily Activities

ACTIVITY/DURATION

Fitness Exercise
Activity for the purpose of health

/

Activities of Living
Physical movement in the daily routine

/

Extra Mile
Intentional physical activity beyond the necessary:
taking stairs, walking vs. transport; standing vs.
sitting; etc.

/

Today I was active for:

___Hour ____ Min

Emoji of the Day

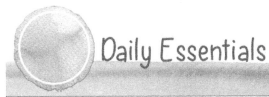

Daily Essentials

Protein First Meals

Protein goal: grams/day

Morning			
PRO	CARBS	FAT	CALORIES
Midday			
PRO	CARBS	FAT	CALORIES
Evening			
PRO	CARBS	FAT	CALORIES
Protein Snack			
PRO	CARBS	FAT	CALORIES

Beverages

Today's Energy Intake
PRO   CARBS   FAT   CALORIES

Obstacle Awareness:
Mindful Preparedness

Daily Activities
ACTIVITY/DURATION

Fitness Exercise
Activity for the purpose of health

/

Activities of Living
Physical movement in the daily routine

/

Extra Mile
Intentional physical activity beyond the necessary: taking stairs, walking vs. transport; standing vs. sitting; etc.

/

Today I was active for:

___Hour ____ Min

Emoji of the Day

Daily Essentials

Protein First Meals
Protein goal: grams/day

Morning				
	PRO	CARBS	FAT	CALORIES

Midday				
	PRO	CARBS	FAT	CALORIES

Evening				
	PRO	CARBS	FAT	CALORIES

Protein Snack				
	PRO	CARBS	FAT	CALORIES

Beverages

Obstacle Awareness:
Mindful Preparedness

Daily Activities
ACTIVITY/DURATION
Fitness Exercise
Activity for the purpose of health

/

Activities of Living
Physical movement in the daily routine

/

Extra Mile
Intentional physical activity beyond the necessary: taking stairs, walking vs. transport; standing vs. sitting; etc.

/

Today I was active for:

___Hour ____ Min

Today's Energy Intake
PRO   CARBS   FAT   CALORIES

Emoji of the Day

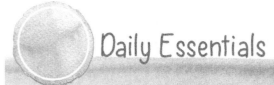 Daily Essentials

Protein First Meals
Protein goal: grams/day

Morning				
	PRO	CARBS	FAT	CALORIES
Midday				
	PRO	CARBS	FAT	CALORIES
Evening				
	PRO	CARBS	FAT	CALORIES
Protein Snack				
	PRO	CARBS	FAT	CALORIES
Beverages				

Today's Energy Intake
PRO   CARBS   FAT   CALORIES

Obstacle Awareness:
Mindful Preparedness

Daily Activities
ACTIVITY/DURATION
Fitness Exercise
Activity for the purpose of health

/

Activities of Living
Physical movement in the daily routine

/

Extra Mile
Intentional physical activity beyond the necessary: taking stairs, walking vs. transport; standing vs. sitting; etc.

/

Today I was active for:
___Hour _____ Min

Emoji of the Day

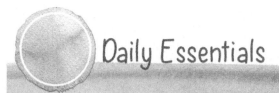

Daily Essentials

Protein First Meals

Protein goal: grams/day

		PRO	CARBS	FAT	CALORIES
Morning					
		PRO	CARBS	FAT	CALORIES
Midday					
		PRO	CARBS	FAT	CALORIES
Evening					
		PRO	CARBS	FAT	CALORIES
Protein Snack					
		PRO	CARBS	FAT	CALORIES
Beverages					

Today's Energy Intake
PRO   CARBS   FAT   CALORIES

Obstacle Awareness:
Mindful Preparedness

Daily Activities
ACTIVITY/DURATION

Fitness Exercise
Activity for the purpose of health

/

Activities of Living
Physical movement in the daily routine

/

Extra Mile
Intentional physical activity beyond the necessary: taking stairs, walking vs. transport; standing vs. sitting; etc.

/

Today I was active for:

___Hour ____ Min

Emoji of the Day

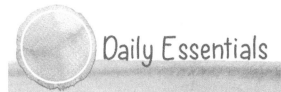 Daily Essentials

Today Is:
S M T W T F S

Protein First Meals
Protein goal: grams/day

Morning	PRO	CARBS	FAT	CALORIES
Midday	PRO	CARBS	FAT	CALORIES
Evening	PRO	CARBS	FAT	CALORIES
Protein Snack	PRO	CARBS	FAT	CALORIES
Beverages				

Today's Energy Intake
PRO   CARBS   FAT   CALORIES

Obstacle Awareness:
Mindful Preparedness

Daily Activities
ACTIVITY/DURATION
Fitness Exercise
Activity for the purpose of health

/

Activities of Living
Physical movement in the daily routine

/

Extra Mile
Intentional physical activity beyond the necessary:
taking stairs, walking vs. transport; standing vs.
sitting; etc.

/

Today I was active for:

___Hour ____ Min

Emoji of the Day

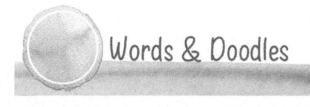

Words & Doodles

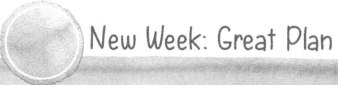

New Week: Great Plan

I've got a good feeling about this!
Week of:

Protein First Meals

Monday	
Tuesday	
Wednesday	
Thursday	
Friday	
Saturday	
Sunday	

Week 11: Goals

Take a small step to improve your health through diet, fitness, and behavior. Add something; eliminate something; change a habit; try something new.
For each category show: ACTION/REWARD

Diet & Nutrition

/

/

Activities of Living

Physical movement in the daily routine

/

/

Fitness Exercise

Activity for the purpose of health

/

/

Notes:

Grocery List

○   ○   ○   ○
○   ○   ○   ○
○   ○   ○   ○
○   ○   ○   Budget $
○   ○   ○   Actual: $

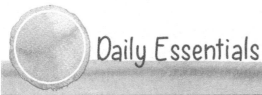 Daily Essentials

Today Is:
S M T W T F S

Protein First Meals

Protein goal: ____ grams/day

Morning				
	PRO	CARBS	FAT	CALORIES
Midday				
	PRO	CARBS	FAT	CALORIES
Evening				
	PRO	CARBS	FAT	CALORIES
Protein Snack				
	PRO	CARBS	FAT	CALORIES

Beverages

Obstacle Awareness:
Mindful Preparedness

Daily Activities
ACTIVITY/DURATION

Fitness Exercise
Activity for the purpose of health

/

Activities of Living
Physical movement in the daily routine

/

Extra Mile
Intentional physical activity beyond the necessary: taking stairs, walking vs. transport; standing vs. sitting; etc.

/

Today I was active for:

____Hour ____ Min

Today's Energy Intake

PRO   CARBS   FAT   CALORIES

Emoji of the Day

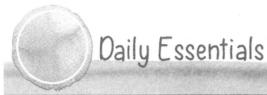

Daily Essentials

Protein First Meals

Protein goal: grams/day

Morning			
	PRO	CARBS	FAT	CALORIES
Midday			
	PRO	CARBS	FAT	CALORIES
Evening			
	PRO	CARBS	FAT	CALORIES
Protein Snack			
	PRO	CARBS	FAT	CALORIES

Beverages

Today's Energy Intake
PRO   CARBS   FAT   CALORIES

Obstacle Awareness:
Mindful Preparedness

Daily Activities
ACTIVITY/DURATION

Fitness Exercise
Activity for the purpose of health

/

Activities of Living
Physical movement in the daily routine

/

Extra Mile
Intentional physical activity beyond the necessary:
taking stairs, walking vs. transport; standing vs.
sitting; etc.

/

Today I was active for:

____Hour ____ Min

Emoji of the Day

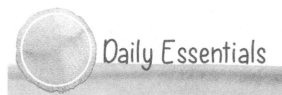

Daily Essentials

Protein First Meals

Protein goal: grams/day

Morning				
	PRO	CARBS	FAT	CALORIES
Midday				
	PRO	CARBS	FAT	CALORIES
Evening				
	PRO	CARBS	FAT	CALORIES
Protein Snack				
	PRO	CARBS	FAT	CALORIES

Beverages

Today's Energy Intake

PRO   CARBS   FAT   CALORIES

Obstacle Awareness:
Mindful Preparedness

Daily Activities

ACTIVITY/DURATION

Fitness Exercise
Activity for the purpose of health

/

Activities of Living
Physical movement in the daily routine

/

Extra Mile
Intentional physical activity beyond the necessary: taking stairs, walking vs. transport; standing vs. sitting; etc.

/

Today I was active for:

___Hour ____ Min

Emoji of the Day

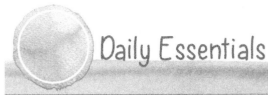 Daily Essentials

Protein First Meals
Protein goal: grams/day

Morning				
	PRO	CARBS	FAT	CALORIES

Midday				
	PRO	CARBS	FAT	CALORIES

Evening				
	PRO	CARBS	FAT	CALORIES

Protein Snack				
	PRO	CARBS	FAT	CALORIES

Beverages

Today's Energy Intake
PRO   CARBS   FAT   CALORIES

Obstacle Awareness:
Mindful Preparedness

Daily Activities
ACTIVITY/DURATION
Fitness Exercise
Activity for the purpose of health

/

Activities of Living
Physical movement in the daily routine

/

Extra Mile
Intentional physical activity beyond the necessary: taking stairs, walking vs. transport; standing vs. sitting; etc.

/

Today I was active for:
____Hour _____ Min

Emoji of the Day

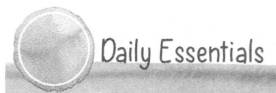

Daily Essentials

Today Is:
S M T W T F S

Protein First Meals
Protein goal: grams/day

		PRO	CARBS	FAT	CALORIES
Morning					
		PRO	CARBS	FAT	CALORIES
Midday					
		PRO	CARBS	FAT	CALORIES
Evening					
		PRO	CARBS	FAT	CALORIES
Protein Snack					
		PRO	CARBS	FAT	CALORIES
Beverages					

Today's Energy Intake
PRO   CARBS   FAT   CALORIES

Obstacle Awareness:
Mindful Preparedness

Daily Activities
ACTIVITY/DURATION
Fitness Exercise
Activity for the purpose of health

/

Activities of Living
Physical movement in the daily routine

/

Extra Mile
Intentional physical activity beyond the necessary:
taking stairs, walking vs. transport; standing vs.
sitting; etc.

/

Today I was active for:
____Hour _____ Min

Emoji of the Day

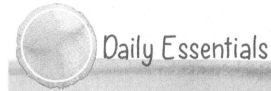
Daily Essentials

Protein First Meals
Protein goal: grams/day

Morning				
	PRO	CARBS	FAT	CALORIES
Midday				
	PRO	CARBS	FAT	CALORIES
Evening				
	PRO	CARBS	FAT	CALORIES
Protein Snack				
	PRO	CARBS	FAT	CALORIES
Beverages				

Today's Energy Intake
PRO   CARBS   FAT   CALORIES

---

*Obstacle Awareness:
Mindful Preparedness*

Daily Activities
ACTIVITY/DURATION
Fitness Exercise
Activity for the purpose of health

/

Activities of Living
Physical movement in the daily routine

/

Extra Mile
Intentional physical activity beyond the necessary: taking stairs, walking vs. transport; standing vs. sitting; etc.

/

Today I was active for:

___Hour ____ Min

Emoji of the Day

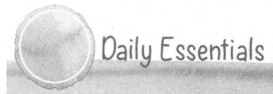 Daily Essentials

Protein First Meals
Protein goal: grams/day

Morning	
	PRO CARBS FAT CALORIES
Midday	
	PRO CARBS FAT CALORIES
Evening	
	PRO CARBS FAT CALORIES
Protein Snack	
	PRO CARBS FAT CALORIES
Beverages	

Today's Energy Intake
PRO   CARBS   FAT   CALORIES

Obstacle Awareness:
Mindful Preparedness

Daily Activities
ACTIVITY/DURATION
Fitness Exercise
Activity for the purpose of health

/

Activities of Living
Physical movement in the daily routine

/

Extra Mile
Intentional physical activity beyond the necessary: taking stairs, walking vs. transport; standing vs. sitting; etc.

/

Today I was active for:

___Hour ____ Min

Emoji of the Day

 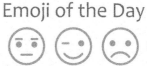

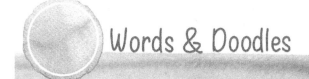

Words & Doodles

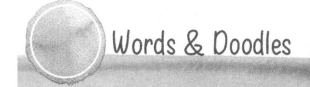

Words & Doodles

New Week: Great Plan

I've got a good feeling about this!
Week of:

Protein First Meals

Monday	
Tuesday	
Wednesday	
Thursday	
Friday	
Saturday	
Sunday	

Week 12: Goals

Take a small step to improve your health through diet, fitness, and behavior. Add something; eliminate something; change a habit; try something new.
For each category show: ACTION/REWARD

Diet & Nutrition
/
/

Activities of Living
Physical movement in the daily routine
/
/

Fitness Exercise
Activity for the purpose of health
/
/

Notes:

Grocery List

○   ○   ○   ○
○   ○   ○   ○
○   ○   ○   ○
○   ○   ○   Budget $
○   ○   ○   Actual: $

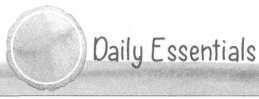

Daily Essentials

Today Is:
S M T W T F S

Protein First Meals
Protein goal: grams/day

Morning				
	PRO	CARBS	FAT	CALORIES
Midday				
	PRO	CARBS	FAT	CALORIES
Evening				
	PRO	CARBS	FAT	CALORIES
Protein Snack				
	PRO	CARBS	FAT	CALORIES

Beverages

Today's Energy Intake
PRO   CARBS   FAT   CALORIES

Obstacle Awareness:
Mindful Preparedness

Daily Activities
ACTIVITY/DURATION
Fitness Exercise
Activity for the purpose of health

/

Activities of Living
Physical movement in the daily routine

/

Extra Mile
Intentional physical activity beyond the necessary: taking stairs, walking vs. transport; standing vs. sitting; etc.

/

Today I was active for:

___Hour ____ Min

Emoji of the Day

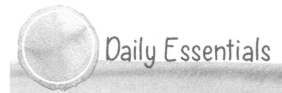

Daily Essentials

Protein First Meals
Protein goal: grams/day

Morning				
	PRO	CARBS	FAT	CALORIES
Midday				
	PRO	CARBS	FAT	CALORIES
Evening				
	PRO	CARBS	FAT	CALORIES
Protein Snack				
	PRO	CARBS	FAT	CALORIES
Beverages				

Today's Energy Intake
PRO   CARBS   FAT   CALORIES

Obstacle Awareness:
Mindful Preparedness

Daily Activities
ACTIVITY/DURATION

Fitness Exercise
Activity for the purpose of health

/

Activities of Living
Physical movement in the daily routine

/

Extra Mile
Intentional physical activity beyond the necessary: taking stairs, walking vs. transport; standing vs. sitting; etc.

/

Today I was active for:

____Hour _____ Min

Emoji of the Day

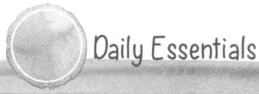

Daily Essentials

Protein First Meals

Protein goal: grams/day

Morning				
	PRO	CARBS	FAT	CALORIES
Midday				
	PRO	CARBS	FAT	CALORIES
Evening				
	PRO	CARBS	FAT	CALORIES
Protein Snack				
	PRO	CARBS	FAT	CALORIES

Beverages

Today's Energy Intake
PRO   CARBS   FAT   CALORIES

Obstacle Awareness: Mindful Preparedness

Daily Activities
ACTIVITY/DURATION
Fitness Exercise
Activity for the purpose of health

/

Activities of Living
Physical movement in the daily routine

/

Extra Mile
Intentional physical activity beyond the necessary: taking stairs, walking vs. transport; standing vs. sitting; etc.

/

Today I was active for:

___Hour ____ Min

Emoji of the Day

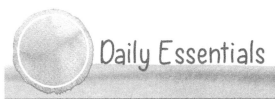 **Daily Essentials**

Protein First Meals
Protein goal: grams/day

Morning				
	PRO	CARBS	FAT	CALORIES
Midday				
	PRO	CARBS	FAT	CALORIES
Evening				
	PRO	CARBS	FAT	CALORIES
Protein Snack				
	PRO	CARBS	FAT	CALORIES
Beverages				

Today's Energy Intake
PRO   CARBS   FAT   CALORIES

Obstacle Awareness: Mindful Preparedness

Daily Activities
ACTIVITY/DURATION
Fitness Exercise
Activity for the purpose of health

/

Activities of Living
Physical movement in the daily routine

/

Extra Mile
Intentional physical activity beyond the necessary: taking stairs, walking vs. transport; standing vs. sitting; etc.

/

Today I was active for:

____Hour _____ Min

Emoji of the Day

Daily Essentials

Protein First Meals
Protein goal: grams/day

Morning				
	PRO	CARBS	FAT	CALORIES
Midday				
	PRO	CARBS	FAT	CALORIES
Evening				
	PRO	CARBS	FAT	CALORIES
Protein Snack				
	PRO	CARBS	FAT	CALORIES

Beverages

Today's Energy Intake
PRO   CARBS   FAT   CALORIES

Obstacle Awareness: Mindful Preparedness

Daily Activities
ACTIVITY/DURATION
Fitness Exercise
Activity for the purpose of health

/

Activities of Living
Physical movement in the daily routine

/

Extra Mile
Intentional physical activity beyond the necessary: taking stairs, walking vs. transport; standing vs. sitting; etc.

/

Today I was active for:

___Hour ____ Min

Emoji of the Day

:) :| ;) :(( )

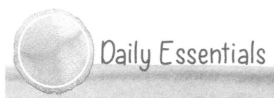

Daily Essentials

Protein First Meals

Protein goal: grams/day

Morning				
	PRO	CARBS	FAT	CALORIES
Midday				
	PRO	CARBS	FAT	CALORIES
Evening				
	PRO	CARBS	FAT	CALORIES
Protein Snack				
	PRO	CARBS	FAT	CALORIES

Beverages

Today's Energy Intake

PRO	CARBS	FAT	CALORIES

---

*Obstacle Awareness:
Mindful Preparedness*

Daily Activities
ACTIVITY/DURATION

Fitness Exercise
Activity for the purpose of health

/

Activities of Living
Physical movement in the daily routine

/

Extra Mile
*Intentional physical activity beyond the necessary:
taking stairs, walking vs. transport; standing vs.
sitting; etc.*

/

Today I was active for:

___Hour ____ Min

Emoji of the Day

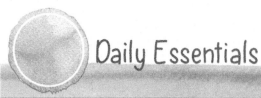 Daily Essentials

Protein First Meals
Protein goal: grams/day

Morning	
	PRO CARBS FAT CALORIES
Midday	
	PRO CARBS FAT CALORIES
Evening	
	PRO CARBS FAT CALORIES
Protein Snack	
	PRO CARBS FAT CALORIES
Beverages	

Today's Energy Intake
PRO   CARBS   FAT   CALORIES

Obstacle Awareness:
Mindful Preparedness

Daily Activities
ACTIVITY/DURATION

Fitness Exercise
Activity for the purpose of health

/

Activities of Living
Physical movement in the daily routine

/

Extra Mile
Intentional physical activity beyond the necessary: taking stairs, walking vs. transport; standing vs. sitting; etc.

/

Today I was active for:
___Hour ____ Min

Emoji of the Day

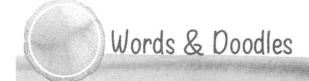

Words & Doodles

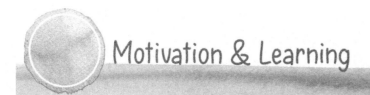

Motivation & Learning

Review of Month 3:

To Do:

Words & Doodles

Words & Doodles

Quarterly Personal Self-Assessment

Date:

The LivingAfterWLS "Quarterly Personal Self-Assessment" tool is a worksheet of questions we can ask ourselves in a sincere effort to assess our present state and make an action plan for the next three months. This worksheet should be used as a private tool with the intent to keep your eye on the goal. It is a contract with yourself; a contract of honor and self-respect because you deserve to treat yourself well and engage in appropriate long-term behaviors in pursuit of your healthiest life. Please accept this invitation to join me in the Quarterly Personal Self-Assessment. Take some quiet time to evaluate where you are and where you are going. Commit your WLS goals to paper. Pre-ops, Newbies and Old-timers all benefit from the use of this tool. You can do this. *Always review your previous quarterly worksheets as you begin this exercise.*

- -

Body: I am physically WELL/ILL *and this is supporting/disrupting my healthy efforts.*

I weigh _____ and I'm [ ] LOSING [ ] GAINING [ ] MAINTAINING.

Mind: I am mentally FOCUSED/DISTRACTED *regarding my WLS experience.*

> *My thoughts are:*

Heart: I am socially and emotionally HAPPY/SAD which is positively/negatively affecting my well-being.

> *My relationships are:*

Write a personal assessment briefly summarizing your overall health and wellness pertaining specifically to your obesity management with weight loss surgery:

My top three goals when I had WLS were:
> Indicate if they are ONGOING (O) CHANGED (C) or ACHIEVED (A)
> 1)
> 2)
> 3)

In pursuit of these goals list the strengths and strategies that are contributing to favorable results:

As with any journey there are struggles. Where have you struggled and what improvements could be made to produce better results?

Define the goal you will pursue this quarter. Why is it important and worthy of your energy and effort? Does it contribute to your long-term health and weight management?

Including your strengths, knowledge, abilities, and intentions define your approach to achieving this goal. Map a strategy for each barrier.

Make a commitment.

Based on the assessment above I will:

The specific tools/methods I will use for my success are:

Will I enlist the help of others? Who/What:

Make your agreement binding:

My next appointment for self-assessment is: _____ (see page 135)

In solemn contract with myself I hereby agree to honor these commitments:

_____

Signature & Date

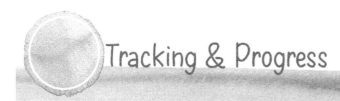

Tracking & Progress

My concerns:

My Motivation:

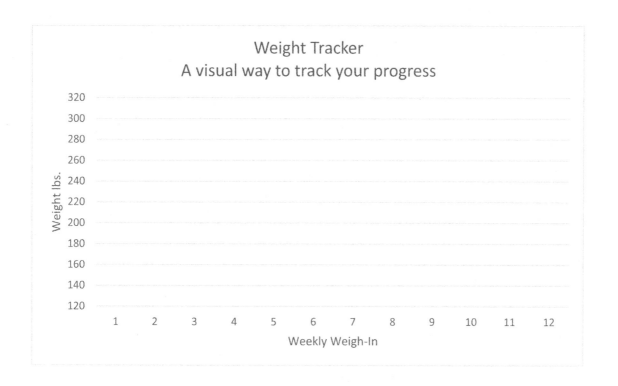

Weight Tracker
A visual way to track your progress

Weight lbs.

| 320 |
| 300 |
| 280 |
| 260 |
| 240 |
| 220 |
| 200 |
| 180 |
| 160 |
| 140 |
| 120 |

1   2   3   4   5   6   7   8   9   10   11   12

Weekly Weigh-In

THE BIG PICTURE:
Based on my Self-Assessment for the next 12 weeks my health and wellness objectives are:

Words & Doodles

Words & Doodles

Words & Doodles

A LIVINGAFTERWLS PUBLICATION

Proudly serving the weight loss surgery community since 2005.

For updates follow me on Amazon
Kaye Bailey's Author Page
https://www.amazon.com/Kaye-Bailey/e/B00LWITO8I/ref=dp_byline_cont_ebooks_1

Made in the USA
Columbia, SC
28 July 2020

14893170R00083